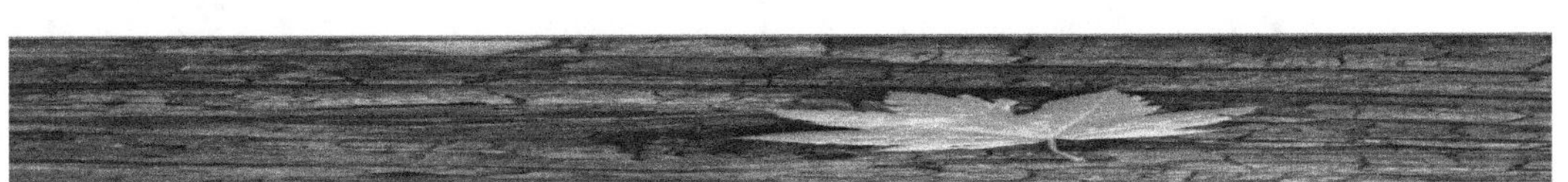

BOOK TITLE: THE WAY TO INNER PEACE

Subtitles: develop your power and thrive

Author: Linda J. Smith

TABLE OF CONTENT

INTRODUCTION..........

CHAPTER 1: What's an HSPS, anyway

CHAPTER 2: How to mention no with out hurting others

CHAPTER 3: A way to keep away from falling in love too quickly

CHAPTER 4: A way to do away with poor energy

CHAPTER 5: A way to filter dangerous partners

CHAPTER 6: A way to cope with stress

CHAPTER 7: Choosing a profession as an HSPS

CHAPTER 8: Thriving at paintings as an HSPS

CHAPTER 9: Parenting as an HSPS

CHAPTER 10: A way to cope with despair as an HSPS

CHAPTER 11: How to triumph over imposter syndrome

INTRODUCTION

Inner peace. It seems like a pipe dream, does't it? How is it possible to find an oasis of calm whilst our lives have ended so busy, stressful, and chaotic?

Inner peace is a country of tranquility in which you feel snug with yourself, others, and the area spherical you. It's about being present and comfortable with your skin. plenty much less impacted through manner of methods of anxiety, worry, and stress.

When you experience inner peace, you get hold of who you are your strengths, flaws, goals, goals everything that makes you uniquely you. You moreover feel more accepting of the area spherical you and the situations which is probably unfolding so you're much less negatively impacted by thru manner method of anxiety, worry, and stress.

This book is majorly approximately excessively touchy humans and the assignments they face and additionally how they can address their surroundings and humans/ courting around them. This book isn't most effectively encouraged for HSPS, even humans who aren't surprisingly touchy can examine it. It includes our daily struggles i.e. depression, anxiety, poor energy, falling in love too quickly, parenting, and additionally imposter syndrome.

Click the buy button now to buy yours.

CHAPTER 1
What is an HSPS, anyway

Have you ever been advised that you're "too touchy" or that you "shouldn't assume so much," mainly with the aid of using individuals who strike you as too insensitive or who you consider must assume a touch more? You can be an exceptionally touchy individual or HSP.

While exceptionally touchy humans are now and again negatively defined as being "too touchy," it's miles a personal trait that brings each strength and challenge.

if you're an exceptionally touchy individual (additionally referred to as HSP), you already know you're without difficulty overstimulated/over-aroused, emotionally touchy and touchy to diffused outside and inner stimuli. You are keenly aware of lights, sounds, smells, and temperature adjustments. You additionally manner your thoughts, feelings, and feelings very deeply, frequently having more potent emotional responses and an eager cognizance of different humans's feelings.

Highly touchy humans are generally very gifted. They feel human connection and like to shape deep bonds and near relationships. They are touchy with different humans's feelings, noticing diffused adjustments in facial expressions or frame language. They generally tend to have vividly practical desires and a standard wealthy internal life.

CHAPTER 2

how to mention no with out hurting others

Saying 'no' can sometimes be tough, can't it?

We often worry about letting people down or upsetting them. But sometimes, saying 'no' is important for our well-being

The trick is not just saying 'no', but how we say it. We need to find a way to say 'no' that does't hurt the other person's feelings.

★ **Be Honest but Gentle**

There's no need to make up excuses if you don't want to do something People appreciate honesty.

However, it's all about how you deliver your message.

★ Knowing how to nicely say "no" is an important part of asserting yourself and setting boundaries. When you constantly say "yes" to things you don't want to do, you may find yourself in challenging situations. When saying "no," there are plenty of ways to reframe your decision politely. By coming off professionally, your coworkers or employer may respect your decision and have a better understanding of your reasoning. As an employee, you have the agency to say "no," but knowing how to do so nicely can make it much easier to do

How to nicely say "no"

Be straightforward.

Instead of saying "maybe" or "I don't think so," be straightforward in your answer. Make sure whoever is asking you the question understands that you mean no now and forever. When you say things like, "maybe later" or "some other time" you should mean what you are saying. Otherwise, these types of in-between answers may prompt the person to ask you the question another time.

Keep your stance

After you say "no," keep that as your final answer. By giving in and changing your answer to "yes," people may be able to get you to eventually agree to things you don't want to do. By staying firm on your answer, your coworkers and employer will understand they can't persuade you any further. It's okay to feel confident about your decision and be in charge of your own life.

Sometimes we need to stop our emotions for good reasons. You can learn how to stop falling in love to avoid getting hurt, but it's better to know how to not fall in love with someone at all!

CHAPTER 3

A way to keep away from falling in love too quickly

Most of us who have a crush on someone end up falling more in love with each passing day.

It's not because we're so helplessly drawn toward that person but because we voluntarily choose to let that person sink their hooks deeper into our hearts. People don't instantly fall in love with the person they like. The feeling you experience is infatuation. And infatuation, as much as it feels like an inescapable wall that blocks your view from everything else, will eventually fade.

You might think that "the heart wants what it wants," and to a degree, yes, it does. But, you can put the brakes on those building emotions and put a stop to any falling in love that may go on. It's possible to learn how to not fall in love with someone, but it takes effort and determination.

Consider if someone is right or wrong for you

If you start to have feelings for someone too soon, you might try to evaluate whether they are right for you or not. Feeling attraction for someone can happen almost immediately, but deeper feelings of love often take longer to develop.

- If you feel like you are constantly falling in "love," try to zoom out and examine the situation objectively to see what you are feeling. Is it love, or is it attraction? One strategy to try to help parse this out may be to consider if the person's qualities and values align with yours and if you two would be a good fit together or not. This may help you regain control of your emotions.
- Focus on other priorities and activities

You may also try to channel the energy that was going toward falling in and out of love into something productive and purposeful. For instance, you could set a new career goal and focus on working towards that.

You could learn a new skill, like playing the guitar or crocheting. You could spend more time with friends or family. Or, maybe you'd like to try a new exercise routine, which can help you stay in shape and give your brain time to rest while doing something beneficial.

 Filling your time with other things you care about may help to keep your frequent romantic feelings in check.

Determine what you're looking for:

Trying some of the strategies above may help you avoid falling in love too quickly with the wrong people, but this does't mean you have to close yourself off from love completely.

- Falling in love with the right person can be a wonderful experience. In addition to the strategies above, it may also help to try to clearly define what you're looking for in a romantic partner and what a healthy relationship looks like for you.

CHAPTER 4

A way to do away with poor energy

Negativity is poisonous for your whole machine, so clearing terrible power is a critical approach to your adventure for internal peace.

Negativity could make you sense heavy, dark, and gloomy; sense emotionally reactive and defensive; and look at the sector via a blended clear out of fear, anger, and paranoia.

MAKE MEDITATION A REGULAR PART OF YOUR LIFE

Spending time inside the stillness of meditation has a profound recuperation impact on the thoughts and facilitates to repairing of your whole machine to stability and positivity. It does this in 3 critical ways.

First, meditation is the antidote to the pressure reaction that's pushed through immoderate awful power. Muscle anxiety is released, blood strain and respiratory are lowered, pressure hormones are minimized, and the fight-or-flight reactivity is down-regulated via meditation.

Secondly, meditation additionally lets you witness your mind as opposed to being stuck up in an interpretation or evaluation.

By witnessing your mind as they arrive and go, you interrupt their move earlier than a terrible interpretation can take root in your intellectual garden.

Thirdly, through again and again moving into the sector of natural consciousness, the terrible opinions on your focus are washed away, freeing their preserve on you.

Like rinsing a dirty cloth in a stream, the negative mental impressions are eventually lifted, returning the cloth to an immaculate state.

GET OUT INTO NATURE

Nature remedy is an effective device to wash the poor electricity out of your thoughts and frame. The purity of nature frequently creates a "device reboot" that facilitates the uninstall of negativity out of your intellectually difficult drive.

When embracing the splendor and majesty of a mountain range, an old-increase forest, the ocean, or the middle of the night famous person field, it will become very hard for poor electricity blocks to hold their preserve in your awareness.

MOVE YOUR BODY

Negative electricity loves inertia and lethargy. Like a black hollow collapsing in on itself, the poor attitude desires to suck you down into oblivion.

One surefire manner to interrupt out of the downward spiral is to rise and circulate your frame. Whether with the aid of doing a little yoga along with Sun Salutations, going for a brisk stroll or run, or some other shape of active movement, vigorously transferring your frame facilitates purging negativity out of your device on numerous levels.

GO COMPLAINT-FREE

Complaining is one of the approaches poor electricity sustains itself in a perpetual movement cycle.

When you're targeted on poor emotions, you whinge approximately matters greater, you pay greater interest to what irritates you, which makes you sense greater poor, and also you whinge again.It's an endless remarks loop of griping and grievances.

The easy fact is this: complaining does't clear up anything. If you've got positive recommendations for the way something may be improved, great. If now no longer, you're best including any other layer to the excess of negativity inside the world.

Chronic complaining is a symptom of a near relative of negativity, and self-pity. It keeps you locked in a perpetual kingdom of "terrible me" and now you no longer have to take duty to your interpretations or how you're feeling.

SMILE OFTEN

Although you might imagine smiling as an easy sentimental or aesthetic activity, there's authentic magic to your smile.

You understand that a grin is contagious to others, however, due to the fact each cell of your frame is eavesdropping on each different cell, a grin isn't localized simply for your face.

Every time you smile, a unique cocktail of neuropeptides is launched that assists in combatting the results of decreased blood pressure and acts as a usual mood-lifter. Naturally, those results make it hard to maintain a poor mood.

CHAPTER 5

A way to filter dangerous partners

Letting go of a relationship is usually not easy. It can be painful to end a relationship even if the relationship was not serving your highest good. Honor any feelings of grief you may have, and allow yourself to feel those emotions rather than attempting to suppress them. Accept grief as a part of the experience, and allow yourself the time you need to heal.

It can be hard to distance yourself from someone you're used to spending so much time with, but it is usually necessary if you want to move on from the relationship. This does't mean you can't maintain a friendship with your ex, but it's usually best to allow some time for both parties to heal before you try to spend time together as friends.

Love often has a way of clouding your perception, which sometimes makes it difficult to see someone for who they are. If you want to get out of an unhealthy relationship, you must be willing to take off your love goggles and look at the person objectively.

It isn't uncommon to only hold on to the good memories of an ex and completely shut out the bad memories. Maintain your perspective by remembering both sides of the experience. Remind yourself of the good times, but don't forget those bad times or you could end up forgetting why you ended the relationship in the first place.

Try your best to shift focus off the relationship and back to yourself.

Consider trying new things or putting your energy into a hobby you've neglected. Remembering why the relationship was unhealthy and focusing on what it is you do want in a relationship can be empowering

Most importantly, work on your relationship with yourself. Focus on cultivating self-love and respect. Remind yourself that you are worthy of love and that you deserve a healthy relationship.

Letting go isn't easy, and it isn't uncommon to forget our own physical and emotional health after a painful breakup. The grief can be overwhelming and we may start to neglect our own needs.

Help yourself by choosing to practice self-care every day. Get plenty of rest. Eat nutritious food. Indulge. Take a hot bath. Get a massage. Whatever it is, just do something to meet your personal needs.

CHAPTER 6

A way to cope with stress

When I communicate "barriers," I imply barriers to your relationships, however I additionally imply it in different approaches as well. This manner turns into greater snug letting humans recognize where you stand and what you want.

When you exercise meditation, you learn how to step again and take a look at your mind and feelings, or even your bodily reactions as separate out of your lifestyles and your "self

Creating "enjoyable zones" can imply having your property be soothing and comparatively freed from conflict. You can accomplish a peaceful surrounding via way of means of including some factors acknowledged to alleviate stress, together with soothing tune and aromatherapy, and having "downtime" there regularly.

Creating calm additionally, manner retaining your near relationships as conflict-loose as possible.

As a notably touchy person, you're probably greater prone to the ravages of sleep deprivation, negative nutrition, and burnout. In this manner you want to make sure to get sufficient sleep at night, four consume wholesome food, and deal with your body, mind, and spirit in something approaches you can.

Practicing self-care will make you greater capable of managing something that comes your way.

Everyone has their specific challenges. As a highly sensitive person, it helps to know what stresses you the most so you can prepare for or avoid those triggers in your life.

CHAPTER 7

choosing a profession as an HSPS

Highly touchy human beings frequently have a deep appreciation for the arts, which makes innovative careers an herbal fit. Careers in artwork, writing, and layout permit HSPs to explicit their sensitivity via their paintings. Whether it is growing stunning visible artwork or crafting evocative stories, HSPs can use their heightened emotional recognition to create paintings that resonate with others.

Many distinctly touchy human beings have a deep choice to assist others. Careers in counseling, therapy, and social paintings permit HSPs to apply their sensitivity to empathize with others and offer support. These professions require emotional intelligence, energetic listening skills, and the potential to hook up with others on a deep level. HSPs excel in those areas, making them perfect for those professions.

Highly touchy human beings frequently have a deep connection to nature and the environment. A profession in environmental or conservation paintings may be distinctly worthwhile for HSPs who are obsessed with shielding the planet. These careers permit HSPs to paint outdoors, in herbal settings, and make an actual effect on the arena around them.

Highly touchy human beings frequently have a sturdy analytical mind, an interest in detail, and a potential to think deeply.

Careers in studies and analysis, inclusive of science, data, and statistics, maybe a wonderful health for HSPs who revel in fixing complicated troubles and digging into data. These careers frequently require operating independently, which may be perfect for HSPs who choose to paint in quiet and centered environments.

For pretty touchy folks who conflict with overstimulation and are crushed in conventional painting environments, entrepreneurship may be a great course. As an entrepreneur, you've got the liberty to create your painting surroundings and set your schedule. HSPs who pick this course can use their sensitivity to become aware of new opportunities, create revolutionary solutions, and construct companies that align with their values and passions.

CHAPTER 8

Thriving at work as an HSP

If you're a pretty touchy individual running with those who don't percentage the trait, it's crucial to embody it.

Being touchy isn't always something you want to cover or make an apology for.

"The excellent decision-makers are frequently folks who are inclined to assume matters through, ask a variety of questions, and take time to talk with the crew and professionals in preference to the short decisive decision-makers that we frequently idolize

extrade the manner you communicate approximately yourself, being open approximately your sensitivity. "It's ok to mention to your manager, 'I'm very touchy with my surroundings, and I do my excellent paintings once I have lengthy durations of recognition without interruptions. What are the right instances in the week that I can timetable that?' That's an affordable question, and it's going to reinforce your overall performance and make a contribution to crew goals."

As a Highly touchy individual, you ought to be aware of your painting's surroundings. Having the potential to do business from home can be perfect as it lets you govern your surroundings and carry out at your complete potential.

If far-off paintings aren't possible, sporting noise-canceling headphones helps, however you could additionally be intentional approximately constructing area into your day

As a touchy person, your mind wishes to technique deeply it won't prevent seeking to do this if you're busy, "For a few people, that is probably scheduling forty minutes or an hour after paintings to simply decompress.

For others, it'd imply doing that in the morning or at a lunch break. Control your environment, especially how you operate some time to construct that area into your life."

CHAPTER 9
Parenting as an HSP

As an extraordinarily touchy character, you could be deeply suffering from pretty much whatever occurs around you, for exact or for ill. The conduct of their friends, own circle of relatives members, and different partners will have a specifically huge impact, which creates a few thrilling demanding situations for HSPs who are lucky sufficient to be parents.

Many extraordinarily touchy humans who've kids are worried that their HSP developments will inhibit their overall performance as mothers or dads. This should no longer happen. An extraordinarily touchy character could make an exceptional discernment if they take the proper technique to the job.

#1 Set limitations that are well-known for your HSP developments.

As an extraordinarily touchy character who's additionally a discern, you want to recognize your limits. Children are often active, demanding, and inquisitive, and they rely upon you to attend to them and generally tend to their maximum critical desires all the time. This will cause them to be a steady presence in your life, and even as you'll typically be extremely joyful to have them around, you ought to recognize that your sensitivities are probably an issue.

When you are taking a private inventory, you can come to comprehend that you're maximum touchy to loud sounds. Or to being touched too often, or to having humans intervene in your private space. Or your tension can be brought about if you're required to carry out too many duties in too brief of a time. Or possibly folks that say impolite or insensitive matters to you could harm you deeply and spoil your day.

Do a number of those observed in your relationships together along with your children? If they do, those conditions must be addressed properly away and adjustments must be made to provide you greater protection.

You should set a few limits and demand that they be respected. Your limitations should be clean and firm, and also you must make certain you've got the distance you require if a number of your children's tough behaviors are herbal and wholesome and shouldn't be curtailed.

#2 Don't deprioritize your needs

Being a figure is the maximum selfless activity someone can have. Your youngsters will continually come first, even after they've grown up and moved out of the house.

All of this means a positive quantity of self-sacrifice. But you shouldn't forget about your maximum essential non-public needs. No matter how busy you become, you need to take time for yourself. You want personal moments wherein you can loosen up and unwind, wherein you can get away from non-stop sensory and emotional stimulation. This is crucial to your intellectual and bodily health, as a fantastically touchy individual you want calm and quiet moments simply as virtually as you want food, water, and air to breathe.

When you are taking time to de-pressure and decompress and accomplish that regularly, your kids will advantage of it simply as an awful lot as you do. You'll be a fantastically touchy figure who can live calm, cool, and collected. You'll continue to be an affected person and could be capable of managing your temper, even in conditions wherein your youngsters' needs and expectancies have left you feeling determined and beaten in the past.

#3. Create an each-day agenda and write down the rules.

Kids may be messy and forgetful. They can also additionally continuously depart matters strewn approximately the residence or of their rooms and by no means trouble to choose them up, even after promising they would. They can also additionally leave their dishes unwashed, the lighting fixtures on after they depart a room, or the fridge door open after they've retrieved a snack.

To alternate this unsettling dynamic, you may strive to matters. One is to create an in-depth written agenda each day, which is the reason for everyone's duties and allows them to understand sure obligations ought to be completed. The second is to make a complete and printable listing of all of the family rules, so your children will understand precisely what's anticipated of them in any respect times. This extra-dependent method of domestic control can assist your kids spoil their complex habits, to be properly for them ultimately and surprising for you each day.

#4. Talk to your kids approximately as a minimum a number of your HSP characteristics.

Many enormously touchy humans suppose they ought to preserve the reality approximately their HSP tendencies to themselves. They can also additionally do this robotically with their youngsters, questioning that it's incorrect to show emotional vulnerability whilst youngsters want dad and mom who're strong, reliable, and responsible. This expertise will assist them in apprehending why you choose to keep away from certain environments, in all likelihood together with a few that they enjoy. It can assist them make changes in their behavior so that they won't do whatever to make you feel crushed or uncomfortable. And possibly maximum importantly, they may usually sense in your direction due to the fact you've depended on them sufficiently to speak in confidence to them approximately your vulnerabilities.

#5. Learn to accept as true with your empathic instincts and allow them to be your guide.

Being an exceedingly touchy individual can create demanding situations whilst you are a parent. But there may be a super upside to being an HSP parent, and in case you cope with matters the proper manner your exceedingly touchy non-public tendencies permit you to forge an extra enjoyable dating together along with your youngsters.

#6. Remain alert for symptoms and symptoms of exceedingly touchy inclinations in your youngsters

if one or more of your youngsters is showing symptoms and symptoms of being an exceedingly touchy individual (and who could be extra certified to identify that than you?), you could be a chief supply of awareness and suggestions for their lives. You can provide sympathy, advice, understanding, perspective, and enlightening tales approximately your very own experiences so that it will assist put together your baby in the existence demanding situations they must face in the years ahead.

#7 Take care of yourself. Just as critical as now no longer pushing yourself is actively looking after yourself. Find an area in which you may rest, do something you enjoy, and retreat into your little world. Some ideas: reading, looking at TV, taking a heat bath, being attentive to music, mendacity down in a dark room, meditating, or praying. You want to take time to decompress and re-energize. Setting apart a while on my own needs to be a part of your everyday routine. Yes, each day.

#8. Accept yourself. Highly touchy humans are brilliant critics and, frequently, perfectionists. They could have issues accepting their flaws and frequently blame themselves for activities of their beyond and present. It's very beneficial to move past the blame via way of means of searching your existence and its demanding situations as a possibility to take action. Ask yourself what a scenario can teach, launch any guilt you have, and consider which you realize the way to circulate forward. Learn your limits. To hold your bodily and emotional well-being, it's miles very critical to set clear obstacles and protect them whilst necessary. You can be tempted to push yourself on your limit, however doing so can include a heavy price, including migraines or continual fatigue.

Pay interest to the diffused messages your frame sends you while you want to return up.

#9. Know that it is ok. Many mothers and fathers sense ambivalence approximately desiring time far from parenting, however, you shouldn't. Separations are right while you and your youngsters are each doing something for yourselves while you are apart. You will go back to your toddler refreshed and extra prepared to revel in being together. Having those varieties of desires no longer makes you "much less than the " right mother and father.

10. Be aware of your thoughts. Highly touchy human beings advantage of a wealthy internal life, however, the disadvantage is they once in a while fear an excessive amount of approximately everything, specifically approximately how others sense. It's difficult to do, however, but if you can keep away from getting stuck in terrible questioning patterns, including fear, regret, and self-blame, it'll decrease your strain and assist you in feeling extra relaxed.

#11. Take parenting breaks. It's easy to turn out to be crushed via way of means of the bodily and emotional needs of kids and the dearth of time to relax. Highly touchy dads and moms want extra time without work from their parenting obligations than different dads and moms do. This calls for mastering a way to ask for assistance and taking common breaks to be by myself and with different adults.

CHAPTER 10
A way to cope with despair as an HSPS

Depression Hits Differently When You're an HSP. Here's How to Handle It.

1. Practice radical self-compassion and deal with yourself with kindness.

Know which you are worthy of treating yourself with the kindness you'll bestow upon an infant or a nice pal, especially while you are going through a depressive episode.

Even while you experience such as you don't have get right of entry for your self-compassion, that's okay, too. In that case, believe what a loving, concerned character for your lifestyle might say to you, and begin from there.

2. Turn to social supports, inclusive of relying on pals or cherished ones who "get" you.

Surrounding yourself with at least some humans and/or cherished animal partners touchy humans have a unique bond with animals anyway! who apprehend and take care of you is critical, especially while you're depressed.

Whenever you are in this state, name your nice pal or own circle of relatives and unashamedly ask them to inform you what they love approximately you, it assists too when you have supportive human beings with the aid of using your facet due to the fact whilst you are feeling low, you want more love and phrases of affirmation.

3. Move your frame, whether or not you pass for a run or do yoga.

Even whilst it feels impossible, befriend and circulate your frame in a manner that receives your coronary heart pumping and makes you experience strong. You may attempt to take a motorcycle ride, take a stroll go for a run across the block, or do yoga poses (mainly warrior ones). Whatever you decide, it's essential sincerely to MOVE. In this manner, you'll assist remodel any poor mind and power into high-quality action.

And if you may get yourself circulate, engage

 in a few radical self-compassion — and consider that you may attempt once more the subsequent day.

4. Try out expressive artwork therapy, like writing, painting, or maybe dancing.

The arts are a safe, contained, and playful manner to specific even the darkest of emotions, and it's far the process, now no longer always the product, that gives the maximum healing. Plus, HSPs are creative, so now's the time to channel that creativity!

Now, at the same time as it's critical to have equipment to locate one's manner through melancholy, it's far similarly critical to create an existence that minimizes melancholy's return. Of course, you can't constantly manage whether or not or now no longer you'll have melancholy, so it's far too high to be aware of the matters you could manage. But right here are some techniques I use to preserve melancholy at bay.

1. Plan something to appear ahead of.

2. Have a nightly mirrored image and gratitude practice.

3. Build a network and connect to different like-minded people.

4. See a therapist or instructor of a few kinds, whether or not it's an existing instruct, a professional instructor, or anything that fits you in high quality.

CHAPTER 11

How to triumph over imposter syndrome

First of all, what's imposter syndrome?

Imposter syndrome is a sense of unworthiness or incompetence, despite attaining accomplishments and success. This feeling is not unusual within the workplace, however, it can happen in much any part of life. Those with imposter syndrome regularly go to brilliant lengths to cover it, which may stunt their destiny success.

1. Know you are now no longer alone

When you've got impostor syndrome, a number of the maximum critical encouragement comes from understanding what number of extremely successful people, each male and female, have constructed extraordinary careers even at the same time as often managing it.

2. Distinguish humility and worry.

There's taking humility on your tough paintings and accomplishments, after which there is feeling conquered with worry due to them. Sometimes, being true to something can cause it to cut the retrofit.

But it's far feasible to experience worth with out feeling entitled, and overcoming impostor syndrome is all approximately locating a healthful stability among the two. Godin is going directly to write, "Humility and worthiness don't have anything in any respect to do with protecting our territory. We ought not to experience like a fraud to additionally be gracious, open, or humble."

3. Let's cross off your internal perfectionist.

Many individuals who are afflicted by impostor syndrome are excessive achievers; individuals who set extraordinarily excessive requirements for themselves and are devoted to doing their pleasant and being the pleasant.

But perfectionism best feeds into your impostor syndrome. When you experience a fud, it is generally due to the fact you are evaluating yourself to a few *perfect* final results it is both not possible or unrealistic.

Not best can no person do the whole lot perfectly, but keeping yourself that widespread may be counterproductive. At a few points, you want to take a step returned and ask yourself: When is right sufficient exact sufficient?

4. Be type to yourself.

Take the stress off yourself and prevent looking to be the professional on day one." advises HubSpot advertising supervisor Jennifer Stafancik.

Impostor syndrome frequently manifests itself as a voice in our heads, berating us with bad messages like "you are now no longer clever enough" or "you are a fraud.

"Negative self-speak is a horrific habit, and it can closely impact our strain and tension levels.

Being typed to yourself" sincerely manner converting the manner you speak to yourself to your head through training superb self-speak. Not handiest can it assist you to be much less burdened and anxious, but it canonically assists you in constructing the braveness to do matters to deliver you more rewards.

First, try and capture yourself on every occasion you've got a bad thought. Then, flip around and venture your claim. For example, in case you discover yourself thinking, "I simply was given luck," venture that through thinking, "What steps did I take and what paintings did I install to get to this point?"

Then, you may solve your query with the usage of affirmations, which are short, focused, superb statements approximately a purpose you've got. In this case, one is probably as easy as "I labored hard – and I continually paintings hard."

5. Track and degree your successes.

When you sense like an impostor, one of the toughest matters to understand is how a whole lot of a position you've got for your successes. You would possibly default them to good fortune or others' difficult work, while, your work, knowledge, and practice had lots to do with it.

To assist display yourself that you are doing well, preserve the tune of your wins in a non-public document.

6. Say "yes" to new possibilities.

It's not possible to say "yes" to everything, in particular, while you are feeling pressured or unfold thin. But it is all too not unusual for humans who've impostor syndrome to show down career-making possibilities due to the fact they do not sense like they have done a terrific job.

When you are provided with a brand new opportunity, it is essential to differentiate between the voice of your head pronouncing you cannot do it due to the fact you are now no longer worth and the only pronunciation you cannot do it due to the fact you've got got an excessive amount of for your plate. The former is your impostor syndrome speaking.

But remember: Taking on tough new paintings and doing nicely at them can open loads of doorways for you. Don't permit your internal impostor to flip down those game-converting opportunities. They can do wonders that will help you learn, grow, and increase your career.

7. Embrace the feeling, and use it.

It's difficult to cast off impostor syndrome completely — especially if you've had it for years and years. The truth that extremely successful humans like "Maya Angelou and Don Cheadle" experience that manner in any case they have performed is proof that it can from time to time be a lifelong condition.

That's why the nice perspective from which to address your impostor syndrome isn't always doing away with it completely; it is preventing it from hindering your success.